Sunbeams Fall

by

Donald M. Ginsberg

ISBN: 1-4033-2336-4 (e-book)
ISBN: 1-4033-2337-2 (Paperback)

Library of Congress Control Number: 2002091491

This book is printed on acid free paper.

Printed in the United States of America
Bloomington, IN

1stBooks - rev. 08/22/02

This book is dedicated to

Joli L. Ginsberg

About the Book

These poems comment on every-day life, with its rapid changes and its frequently amusing peculiarities and paradoxes. Over half of the poems are humorous, but many are serious. Almost all have regular rhyme and meter. The poems implicitly express the author's philosophy of life: enjoy our beautiful universe (it's the only one we've got), share a laugh, and try not to stub a toe on every passing chair.

Have you ever had a computer ask you for a date, or tell you that you are deceased? Have you ever fallen in love in a laundromat? Do you find it hard to get going in the morning? Are you amused by people who make too many excuses, or who sing off key? Do you love rocks or mountains or quirky friends? Have you wondered what to do with your retirement years? Then this book is for you.

Contents

Preface

With one exception, these poems were written in the years following the author's retirement in August, 1997. He has set several of these poems to music.

Joli L. Ginsberg, the author's wife and best friend, has been helpful in reacting sensitively to these verses. This book is dedicated to her.

Donald M. Ginsberg
Urbana, Illinois
March 20, 2002

<u>Serious Remarks</u>

A Poet Speaks

A poet speaks, but we must hear the sound,
And how are we to hear a voice unknown?
Poets now with greenest laurel crowned
Were unfamiliar once, and all alone.

The humble poet, with his dreams of fame,
Possesses little but the ink, just dry
On pages that he hopes will bring his name
To some with help to give and friendly eye.

How did Poe and Shelley first resound,
E. B. Browning, Alexander Pope,
T. S. Eliot, Byron, Whitman, Pound,
Or Tennyson, when all they had was hope?

These and other poets paid to see
Their works displayed for us by their own hand.
Likewise, you see these verses, launched by me
In hopes they'll find a tender spot to land.

When I'm with You

When I'm with you and hold your hand so warm,
The sky is blue, though thunder clouds may swarm.
The sun may hide, and winter winds may blow;
You light it all with summer's fairest glow.

When you're with me and whisper in my ear,
You're all I see, though sun-drenched clouds are near.
Though glowing skies may paint the world with fire,
Your sparkling eyes my deepest love inspire.

When you're away and time creeps slowly by,
I see no day, though clouds depart the sky.
Though sunbeams fall and bring their light to me,
Dark night is all my weeping eyes can see.

The golden sky may change to gray or blue;
The world I see depends on only you.

A Book

A book is a wonderful thing.
Its author should feel like a king.
With its words it can teach
Even those out of reach
How to live, and to prosper, and sing.

The symbols we see on the pages
Exhibit the concepts of sages,
And the type, set with care,
Makes the reader aware
Of a beauty that's stored for the ages.

Sweet Are Shouted Words

Sweet are shouted words of praise,
Sweeter are the quiet days that follow.
If forest murmurs still amaze
And falling leaf can fix your gaze tomorrow.

Donald M. Ginsberg

Great Composers

Great composers, long departed,
Sing through me.
The magic of the paths they charted
Set me free
To touch and move the tenderhearted
Gratefully.

Euclid's Child

I praise you, pregnant pentagon,
Among the shapes, a paragon,
Replete with possibilities,
Empowered by your symmetries,
Discerned in Grecian days of old,
Delighting eyes as you unfold
The fascinating bold designs
Implicit in your graceful lines.

Though eyes may fail and books may burn,
To your fine form I shall return
With inward sight again to see
Your beauty, stored in memory;
And when I've gone beyond the sky,
Then others will your splendor spy;
You wait for them with charm to show,
More fair than outward sight can know.

Donald M. Ginsberg

Ode to a Rock

Behold this messenger upon my shelf,
Bringing to my gaze a hint of forces
Deep inside the earth in ancient days,
Molten rock in fiery fiercest flow
Or silent transformations, pressed so hard,
Or slow accretion, aged beyond our thoughts.
Row on row, layer forming layer,
Building facets in the darkest depths,
Never dreaming of the future day
When light would dance and bend and sometimes bounce
To fill my eye with colored forms, and hint
Of nature's deepest laws, the ancient truths.
Behold this silent rock with tales to hear
Of ancient days and laws and beauty clear.

I Slumbered in a Seminar

I slumbered in a seminar and dreamed of streets of gold,
Where manuscripts were strewn about with wisdom to unfold.
Each was so significant that it could win a prize,
Delighting friends and colleagues, bringing joy beyond
    disguise.

I dreamed of marble halls in which experiments were done,
All of them successful and without a wasted run.
Alas, I was awakened when a bell began to peal;
I came back to my senses in a place that's all too real.

If Pen Could Scribe

If pen could scribe or voice exclaim
Your beauty or your worth,
I would not rest until your fame
Were spread throughout the earth.

Survival

When night-clouds thunder, I often wonder
At nature's awesome might;
And how could Neolithic man
Survive on such a night?

When winter's hand engulfs the land
And blankets all in snow,
I ask myself: How did those tribes
Survive 'til spring-time's glow?

Donald M. Ginsberg

For This I Hold You Dear

For this I hold you dear:
Your attitude;
You judged what you did hear
With latitude.
Your kindness draws a tear
Of gratitude.
"Thank you" seems, I fear,
A platitude;
So let me wish you here
Beatitude.

A Quiet Man

I met a man from a town so small,
It wasn't on the map at all;
Not even billboards steered you to the place.
The man seemed square, without a care.
His ancestors had settled there
For reasons that were lost without a trace.

You could walk around and not go wrong:
The only street was one block long,
With nothing but a dog to block your way.
Throughout the lazy afternoon,
By the shaded door of the town's saloon,
The dog would sleep and dream the hours away.

Go discover such a town.
Find a friend to ask you down,
And pay a little visit to the place.
Take the time to stay a while,
Fall into the quiet style,
And tune your nervous system to the pace.

Unheeded

Out where winds are unimpeded,
Oft I've gone to sing unheeded,
Shouting out my pain with none to hear.
None to witness words of sorrow
Or the notes I humbly borrow,
None to see the falling of a tear.
Then, my thoughts from where I'm singing
Drift away, so gently winging
To the one I love, though far away.
As I see her in my mind,
My tangled thoughts somehow unwind,
And peaceful feelings all my fears allay.

When I Was Young

When I was young, and you along with me,
The moon would rise and send its light to see,
Its moonbeams falling on your tender face.
Of all the earth, this was my lucky place.

When you are old, and I along with you,
The sun of gold will pierce the icy blue,
And fall upon your head, so dear to me,
Resplendent beauty for my eyes to see.

The Gray of Winter

The gray of winter settles on the land;
The woods are dimly lit by grazing beams.
Early sunsets tell of snow to come
And fall upon the frozen ponds and streams.

Winds that blow across the rutted roads
Scatter leaves that fell and piled up deep.
From barren trees the birds have flown away.
And beasts of fields will soon be fast asleep.

The gray of winter creeps into my soul,
Whispering the loss of sunny day.
In solitude, my voices call to me;
They say "Soon you will also fade to gray."

Red Herring, Red Herring

Red Herring, Red Herring, what have you caught
In your net, called a workshop for poets assorted?
You've caught an old fish, but the look on his face
Seems to say that your fisherman's hopes are aborted.

His lips do not smile, his eyes do not sparkle,
His voice seldom rises, his joy he conceals;
And yet he informs you he writes funny verses,
And borrows your face to express what he feels.

Permit me to help you explain what you're seeing.
Just pay close attention, and lend me your eyes.
On the fish's bent shoulders, you'll see something crouching,
Its name you must guess if you're claiming the prize.

This burden has crouched on the backs of the famous,
A fighter who dances and stings like a bee,
The pope in his church, hardly able to mutter,
It's a devil named Parkinson there that you see.

When the face of the fish isn't smiling or laughing,
Try to remember to think of your own.
He's using your face to display his emotions,
Since his is impassive, as when he's alone.

Donald M. Ginsberg

For a Laugh

Donald M. Ginsberg

A Poet's Lament

Night again descends upon my mailbox.
Another day is gone, with all my dreams.
My book's first draft, which flew to you last week,
Languishes in darkness and in chains.
I hope some day to see it on display
In Dallas, San Francisco, Mandalay:
Stacks of books, arranged and rearranged,
Craving the embrace of loyal fans
Who stand with racing hearts on quiet feet,
Noses pressed against the windowpanes,
Slowly shifting toward the open door
Until they, too, can squeeze into the store

A Singer's Dreams

I am never forgetting the day
When my teacher is pausing to say
That I have a good voice, and therefore a choice,
Because singing could bring me some pay.

He wants me to visit the Met;
An appointment for me he can get.
If I pass my audition, I'll be in condition
To prosper and get out of debt.

I will prance up and down on the stage,
Adulation and love I'll engage.
They will cheer me for hours and throw me some flowers;
In the newspapers, I'll be the rage.

The girls will see my good looks,
They will bring me their autograph books.
They'll beg for a chance to persuade me to dance;
Into me they'll be getting their hooks.

I hope I am not only dreaming;
Opportunities vast I am scheming.
Perhaps a good start would be taking to heart
The advice that calls practice redeeming.

Donald M. Ginsberg

Halted on the Interstate

Halted on the Interstate,
Trucks to left and right,
Another one in front of you,
Blocking out the sight
Of hills and streams and meadows green,
The things you'd hoped to see
This morning when you filled your car
And set out eagerly.

Welcome to your traffic jam,
We hope you've got all day.
We trust you've brought some songs and cards
To wile the hours away,
But tunes and tricks turn tedious
While trapped in traffic's tide;
You'll curse the day you ventured forth
Without a horse to ride.

The Hills of Urbana

When I climb up Yankee Ridge and gaze across the fertile
    fields
To the distance where the prairie meets the sky,
I am struck by all the beauty of the gently rolling hills,
You can see them with a keen Urbana eye.

Memories

Allow me to present to you
This person, whom I know,
Whose name I have forgotten,
Though I learned it long ago.

I hope you'll get to be his friend,
Sharing games and chores;
Then you can tell his name to me
When I've forgotten yours.

The Voice

Once I lived alone, and was as lonesome as a star.
Pairing with a woman was my strongest wish by far.
"The wish is father to the thought," a wise man once
    proclaimed,
And thinking of a woman caused my heart to race untamed.

My phone rang just at midnight, and it whispered in my ear,
Expressing admiration and addressing me as "dear,"
Suggesting that we have a date to deepen our relation,
Entreating me to choose a mode of joyous dissipation.

She began to give me options for the way we should proceed:
"Push 1 for conversation, and push 2 for other need."
I was hearing a computer; it was not a living girl!
I hung up and began to cry; my mind was in a whirl.

"I'm going to buy a paper doll," a poet once declared,
But cyber love won't satisfy my longing to be paired.

We're Sorry

We're sorry our computer indicates you are deceased,
And you've bolted with no forwarding address.
We see our records show that all your files were released
And were published in the scandal-making press.

We'll gladly fix our records if you'll only.pay your dues,
Though we seldom take a payment from the dead.
We will notify the media that you no longer choose
To be a self-confessed abuser who has fled.

If this response is helpful, we are programmed to be glad,
And we'll eagerly address your future needs.
Please count on us and be assured; you shouldn't feel so bad,
Because we back up all the files of your misdeeds.

Pianissimo Don

Pianissimo Don is known hither and yon
As a flutist who never plays forté.
Though he gives it his best at his teacher's behest,
He is always found coming up shorté.

With unstable staccatos, unsteady legatos,
Key signatures lost in the fray,
You can never be sure what you'll have to endure,
Once he commences to play.

When you witness his phrasing and glitches amazing,
You'll wish he would leave you alone.
But if those seem bad, then just listen a tad
To his tonguing and tuning and tone.

So head for the hills to escape from his trills,
His vibrato and high notes, all tight,
And pray for the day when they'll finally say
"With his flute he has vanished from sight."

Donald M. Ginsberg

Many a Flute

Many a flute has met its end
When someone sat upon it.
A sadder tale has ne'er been penned,
In history or sonnet.

A music stand is close at hand,
A tempting resting place
To put the flute while it is mute,
But it may fall apace.

So never put your flute away
Upon a chair or music stand,
Unless you have the urge to play
The flattest notes in all the land.

Scenarios for Retirement

I need a physics book, I need a quiet nook,
I need a pad and pencil by my side.
I need an easy chair without a care
So my mind can be applied.
Then my eyes will fill with equations 'til
I've gained some understanding
Of the world I see, the way it ought to be,
With the order that my soul's demanding.

I need a small PC, I need a big TV,
I need a coffee cup by my side.
I need to see the Web or hear what's said
While the caffeine takes me for a ride.
With a zapper I can surf all over the turf,
With a mouse I can reject or choose;
I control my world, my power's unfurled,
Without the need for booze.

I need a flute, I need a fiddle, a piano in the middle,
Musicians by my side.
I need a music stand, I need a score in hand,
My joy I would not hide.
With Mendelssohn or Mozart we'll move along,
Shaping every note and pause,

Donald M. Ginsberg

(Continued)

Into a gigue we'd slowly lead
Expecting some polite applause.

I need a pickup truck, I need a can of beer,
I need a girlfriend by my side.
I need a dog, I need a map, I need a baseball cap;
I'm gonna take 'em for a ride.
We'll bounce along with a whoop and a song,
Kicking up a cloud of dust,
Tossing our trash on the highway,
Proud of our noise and rust.

Statistics

I've studied probability, although my brain's debility
Has slowed me down and made my progress hard.
With every problem solved, I have found myself involved
In conundrums that have put me on my guard.

From arguments statistical, conclusions that are mystical
And other strange results have seemed to follow.
So please allow me to present some odd conclusions that are
    meant
To teach us things we'll find it hard to swallow.

Watch some games of basketball; then you'll know it makes
    you tall,
And meals in fancy restaurants make you rich.
Hospitals, for all their skill, apparently make patients ill,
And being dirty puts you in a ditch.

Donald M. Ginsberg

The Broker

When you get your margin call,
Your blood is turned to ice.
He says it's not his fault at all,
Just blame it on the dice.
But when the market roars ahead,
And your stocks soar like a bird,
He surely blames himself instead,
Although it seems absurd.

Gables

Of gables too many, my thoughts for a penny
I'll offer, if only you'll listen:
I prefer a design with an elegant line,
From which everything excess is missin'.

I freely confess I'm addicted to mess,
But not where my neighbors can see.
I prefer my debasement confined to my basement,
Where it's visible only to me.

Rhymester

A man who puts thoughts into rhyme
Shouldn't do it too much of the time.
He's apt to converse
With an excess of verse;
He'd do better if he were a mime.

CAT Scan, Myelogram

CAT scan, myelogram, EKG,
I don't know who's doing them, but they sure know me.
They've looked at every organ and they've imaged every
    bone;
Now all I ask is: Go away and leave me alone.

You prodded and you poked me with your miracle machines;
Now you want to cut me with your swords and guillotines.
You can take your bloody bandages and keep your awful food;
Go operate on someone else, I'm not in the mood.

Once When I Was Young

Once when I was young, I was an early-morning guy.
I'd leap from bed to greet the day as dawn lit up the sky.
With eager steps I'd hunt around for useful things to do,
So lunch-time's call would follow a completed task or two.

But now I sleep well past the dawn, and in my bed I stay.
My body doesn't activate 'til later in the day.
Yet, while the sun still climbs the sky, I have my dressing
    done,
So I can say without a lie, "I'm up before the sun."

Waiting

I don't know when I came here,
Can't remember that far back.
My prearranged appointment's
For a time long gone, alack.
The fellow's nowhere to be seen,
I hope he's on the job.
Otherwise, my wait could last
'Til hair grows on my knob.

I'll be here 'til the stars burn out,
'Til none recalls Babe Ruth.
'Til butterflies can butter toast,
And Lincoln shoots John Booth.
'Til water runs uphill in June
And clouds are red and green,
'Til heat can flow from cold to hot,
And purple pigs are seen.

Donald M. Ginsberg

For You I'd Gladly

For you I'd gladly write a verse,
Because you ask so nicely,
But I haven't time 'cause it's got to rhyme,
And every line has to have the right number of syllables.

No Jelly Bean

No jelly bean shall pass these wayward lips,
Nor piece of pie nor cake nor any sweet
'Til I have taken weight from off my hips,
Restoring my old shape without retreat.

No foods like these, when put before my eyes,
Shall find their way past teeth into my gut,
Nor will they sneak aboard like lowly spies
While brain's in deepest sleep and eyes are shut.

More forcefully than Hamlet, that poor soul,
Planning with more foresight than King Lear,
Abandoning stout Falstaff as my role,
Like Cassius, lean and hungry I'll appear.

With this, my warfare on the jelly bean,
I now begin my struggle to be lean.

Donald M. Ginsberg

I'm Spooked by Volatility

I'm spooked by volatility,
It's stolen my stability
And driven all my thoughts around the bend.
The market's got me spooked for sure;
It's more than patience can endure
And makes me wonder, where's it all to end?

With a daily dance of death, the Dow
Defies our wildest thoughts, and now
The NASDAQ takes its heart-arresting leaps.
The spectacle of wild gyration
Soon will force me to vacation
Somewhere far away from broker's beeps.

I Got My New York Times

I got my New York Times,
I got my songs and rhymes,
I got my girl friend by my side,
I am just as happy as I can be.

I got my small PC,
I got my big TV,
And my books take me for a ride,
I am just as happy as I can be.

    Among life's pleasures,
    These are the best,
    They can't be measured,
    They can only be blessed.

I got the sun in the sky,
I got a twinkle in my eye,
My joy can't be denied,
I am just as happy as I can be.

Donald M. Ginsberg

Rocks

There are rocks that show you sparkles that delight the human
   eye,
And rocks whose lovely facets lift your spirits to the sky.
There are purple rocks and yellow rocks that captivate your
   heart,
And rocks whose surface structures show the best of nature's
   art.

But rocks are very special in a more important way:
They're absolutely faithful; where you put them, they will
   stay.
They never say sarcastic things, or try to take your place;
Of jealousy or rancor they will never show a trace.

So raise your glass and join my toast to reassuring friends:
The rocks that rest upon our shelves while none of them
   offends.
You can take your dogs and kittens and the hamsters that you
   meet.
My pets are rocks; they bring to me a happiness complete.

Confidence

I'm sure we'll be acquitted, for our case will be appealed.
We wouldn't be in trouble now if Joey hadn't squealed.
The story that the papers told was taken out of context.
If the public knew us better, there would surely be no contest.

We never did those awful things the cops accuse us of.
We thought we'd be protected when we threw away the glove.
We promise we will never do those dreadful things again,
So it's all quite clear, please be a dear, don't send us to the
    pen.

Donald M. Ginsberg

Confusion

Dermatologists treat ailments that afflict the human hide,
And internists cure problems of the parts one finds inside.
That much is clear, but still, I fear, confusion may ensue:
For all the other doctors, what is left for them to do?

Pills

There are pills for all the aches and ills that medicine can treat,
Pills of every size and shape, and hue,
To sort the pills each morning is an effort to complete.
And you wonder: is the outcome good for you?

There are pills to make you happy, there are pills to make you
    calm,
There are pills to help you when you want to sleep.
There are pills that can destroy you just as surely as a bomb,
There are pills that almost make you want to weep.

There are pills that go directly to a sore and stiffened joint.
How do they know where they're supposed to go?
They can cure a head that's throbbing and they never
    disappoint,
Whether needed near your top or down below.

Whatever is your problem, pills can help put it behind you,
And there's hardly any need they cannot fill.
But the pill that we are lacking is the one that would remind
    you
When the time has come to take another pill.

Donald M. Ginsberg

A Second Opinion

When you hear your doctor's voice
Pronouncing that you're dead,
Remember that you have a choice:
Ask someone else instead.

A Short Story

On a lucky day I won't forget,
I met her in a launderette.
I found her graceful as a feather.
Now we wash our clothes together.

Donald M. Ginsberg

Daunting

His Dante is daunting, his Flaubert he's flaunting,
He quotes Heinrich Heine all day.
But why he so seldom will speak for himself,
I am simply unable to say.

Old songs by Scarlatti and more by Menotti
He sings with a voice that is fine,
But often a song whose composer's long gone,
Eternally still and supine.

I Sold My Soul

I sold my soul on eBay to a guy they call the Devil.
Then I found, to my dismay, he wasn't on the level.
Only banks in Hell can cash the check with which he paid,
And thus, until I die, no compensation will be made.

Donald M. Ginsberg

Please Don't Tell My Friends

Please don't tell my friends I died at Wal-Mart.
Say I died at Tiffany's or Saks.
I never buy accessories at Hallmark,
And I hope I'm never seen at T. J. Maxx.

I will bargain with a salesman as I lie upon a stretcher,
While the rescue squad removes me from the store,
Where my ghost will still appear, showing how to persevere,
Seeking sales throughout the year forever more.

Airplane Travel

Airplane travel, so they say,
Is a trip through friendly skies,
But sometimes, on your travel day,
It proves quite otherwise.

When airport lines are a mile long,
And the clerks are throwing fits,
You'll wonder why things go so wrong
That you almost lose your wits.

When the flight you need becomes delayed
And they cancel your connection,
And they've chosen you to be displayed
In their most complete inspection,

You're bound to wish your trip by flight
Were just a hike instead,
And you'll pray to God that the Brothers Wright
Had simply stayed in bed.

Donald M. Ginsberg

So Long

So long, you ancient pitch; I go my way.
Because I sing off tune, I cannot stay.
But if some day by chance the key I find,
Your sound will not be very far behind.
Until that day, the note will come out flat,
And friends will have to pardon me for that.

Weight Watching

My doctor says to watch my weight.
On this my health depends,
And so I watch it carefully;
I see that it ascends.

The Cat

Beware the noble wild cat,
Dreaded in his habitat.
Avoid this horrifying beast,
Lest he see you as his feast.
Shun this speedy adversary
Whose teeth and claws are legendary.

kitty cat
kitty cat
kitty cat cat

cat kitty
cat cat
kitty

Tax Man

Figuring out your income tax
Is a daunting task indeed.
Forms galore you've got in store,
To do with skill and speed.
And as you slog through the tax-man's swamp,
This rule is good, you'll find:
Though the tax man mines your savings,
You must try to save your mind.

Donald M. Ginsberg

I Want to See a Mountain

I want to see a mountain, and I want to see it now.
We've crossed the State of Kansas, and my wife has made a
    vow
Nevermore to make this trip in our trusty Chevrolet
Until they rotate Kansas, and we cross the shorter way.

Sometimes I Am Driven Mad

Sometimes I am driven mad
By interruptions I have had
From mail delivered to the door,
With more demands, forever more.

See my desk's majestic flow
Of glaciers carrying not snow,
But bills and notices abounding,
Catalogues in stacks astounding.

Sometimes when I contemplate
How to slow the torrent's rate,
There's a thought I can't resist:
I'd hate to find I'd not been missed.

Spaghetti

Spaghetti comes out best when cooked
With basil and a scallion,
Just like Grandma would have made
If she had been Italian.

Speeding Down the Highway

Speeding down the highway
With my Joli at the wheel,
Scattering chickens left and right,
Hear those tires squeal.

She's not in fear of trucker guys
In their monster truck machines,
Or the way they shout and wave to her
In their caps and faded jeans.

She refers to herself as "little old me,"
But truckers fear her name.
Once they've seen this driving machine,
They're never again the same.

Eat your hearts out, trucker men,
As she shows you how to drive.
Tell the folks when you're home again:
This legend is still alive.

Donald M. Ginsberg

<u>Physics Observations</u>

Donald M. Ginsberg

The Laws of Physics

Our universe, with its display,
Delighting us by night and day,
In mathematical accord
Evolves by statutes of the Lord.

Dedicated to Eugene Hirsch,
physician, musician, and poet.
His hands heal human hearts.

Oscillations Electromagnetic

Oscillations electromagnetic
I send you with signals of love,
Generated by motions frenetic
Of electrons, by laws from above.
The message flies on as by magic
At velocity none can exceed.
If my meaning were lost, 'twould be tragic;
Let no one my signals impede.

Donald M. Ginsberg

Circuits

I close my eyes and sing of circuits,
Wires forming highways for the flow of charge.
I see electrons sailing freely on the Fermi sea,
Buoyed up by the Pauli principle.

I envision matter-waves diffracted by the crystal lattice,
Bragg-reflected, particles leaping through reciprocal space.
Blessed are the boundaries of the Wigner-Seitz cell;
Thank you, Lord, for constructive interference.

I dream of surface states on chips abounding,
Charge carriers lurking in classically forbidden regions.
The tails of wave functions piercing barriers,
The tunneling of Cooper pairs, energy without entropy,

How sweet, to contemplate the signals so produced,
Flying forth on wings of Faraday!

The Quantum Hall Effect

The Quantum Hall Effect has shown
That lovely nymphs arise full grown
From ordinary woodland ponds
Or from some lowly garden fronds.

Whoever would have guessed that Hall,
By means that weren't complex at all,
Had found a bud which, when unfurled,
Would change the way we view the world?

Albert Einstein

Albert Einstein doesn't live here any more.
You won't find him, though you search the planet o'er.
He has left us all alone, and we wish we had his clone,
Because he changed our way of thinking to the core.

Quantum Secrets

There's a secret little booklet, it's as handy as can be
When you're thinking of the properties of things too small to
  see.
The gurus have a copy, but they keep it to themselves,
And they never leave it carelessly on chairs or desks or
  shelves.

Heisenberg's uncertainty drives students to the brink,
And the famous cat of Schrödinger can claw them 'til they
  sink.
Collapsing coefficients make them run away in fright.
Entangled states tie minds in knots that bind them day and
  night.

That nonsense taught to students has absurdities to swallow,
And a swamp full of confusion where the unanointed wallow.
The gurus hide the wisdom that the booklet's lines display,
Except to those who shake their hand in a secret kind of way.

So if you want to understand a very little thing,
Like an atom, an electron, or a photon on the wing,
Don't bother to peruse again the books that you despise;
Just learn the guru's handshake, and he'll open up your eyes.

Donald M. Ginsberg

<u>Some Friends</u>

Donald M. Ginsberg

Ehud Yairi

Ehud Yairi can make you feel cheery
While searching for money to pay
For the poor and arthritic or projects Semitic
From funds you have salted away.

You will give him your thanks as he empties your banks
And the hiding place under your bed
You will praise him for taking the dough you've been making,
Not noticing how you've been bled.

So when he comes calling, there's no use in stalling,
Be sure to remain on your guard;
Lock all of the doors, get down on all fours,
And hide while he waits in the yard.

But, though you have needs, if you find he succeeds
And he pries all your cash boxes loose,
At least you will know, as to poor house you go,
That your dough will be put to good use.

Linda Ginsberg

Above the clouds, beyond our caution's plead,
Where none but birds and mountain goats should go,
Down she swoops with ever greater speed
Past pine trees, through the madly flying snow.
With graceful form, her poles slash swift and bold.
With rhythm sure she swerves from left to right,
A blur of motion, wild but controlled,
Has ever there been such a sparkling sight?

Donald M. Ginsberg

Doctor Kenneth Aronson

Doctor Kenneth Aronson,
On whom we all depend,
Keep us, by comparison,
In shape until our end.

To keep your expert skills engaged
And pique your curiosity,
We'll hope for symptoms real, not staged,
That challenge virtuosity.

Laura Greene

Here's to the winner of prizes so many,
As famous as Bernstein (the one they call Lenny).
Your friends all delight at the beautiful sight,
And your prizes should quiet your critics (if any).

Donald M. Ginsberg

Jack Stillinger

Jack Stillinger, we bid you rise
With all your former might.
Your friends won't rest until their eyes
Have feasted on the sight.

Ed Dessen

Ed Dessen gave me sound advice;
He didn't have to say it twice:
Even though your surgeon's able,
Pause before you mount his table.
The knife he wields could do the worst,
So ask another doctor first.

Virginia Metze

We have witnessed wondrous ways,
Prompting us to pause and praise:
Here's to Metze's mighty minions,
Mending our computing engines,
Zapping zealously, these heroes,
All the wayward ones and zeroes,
Righting wrongs in record time
With secret cyber skills sublime.

Anthony J. Leggett

There's a Tony, a saint, who helps find lost possessions;
There's a Tony who leads at the Commons's sessions.
A Tony who bounces and says things are Grrreat!
And a Tony for actors to show they're first-rate.
But our Tony, whose thinking has earned highest praise,
His way of doing physics can only amaze.

Elizabeth Klein Shapiro

Enormous pride thou mayest in us behold,
Since we have seen a poet in our gates
With strokes of pen a wondrous book unfold,
And sell it in the big-time market place.
This self-same poet taught our Sunday school,
Illuminating minds where dark did dwell,
And reading to us with a mellow voice
That stirred our hearts, and caused our tears to well.
Where is thy pride, New York, from which we gained
This noble soul, this four-fold mother too?
Why weepst thou England, that she graced thy shores
So short a time with bearded friend and true?
Be sure of this: That though her name is Klein,
She has grown mighty, and enriched our time.

John Bardeen

Thank you, Lord, for John Bardeen,
And for the many things we've seen
With help from minds of depth and vision,
Back to ancient Greek precision.

Thank you, Lord, for everything
Of which, each day, our spirits sing;
But most of all, our voices rise
In thanks for inner vision's eyes.

Donald M. Ginsberg

Miles Klein

Miles writes papers that light up the world,
And teaches his classes with brilliance unfurled.
For a physics professor with research and teaching,
His wardrobe is splendid, and suited for preaching.
He interprets his data with light from above,
And makes funding officers coo like a dove.
He leads complex efforts of folks temperamental,
And soothes jangled nerves, lest they grow detrimental.
Though his last name is Klein, which in German means small,
His concepts are large, and his textbook stands tall.
When a crisis arises, demanding a pro,
We all feel secure when we've Miles to go.

Paul Goldbart

Goldbart's name means beard of gold,
But now we know he's gotten old,
Forty years, to be exact,
With a mind that's still intact.
I'm happy for him on this day,
Though his beard is turning gray.

Donald M. Ginsberg

Lizey Goldwasser

I found a rare treat, bringing joy that's complete,
In the town of Urbana one day:
A poet named Lizey, with poems so lively,
She'd blow William Shakespeare away.

Harold Gluskoter

No wonder Leah likes this guy,
He's quick as he can be,
And pleasant, deep, and sensitive,
As anyone can see.
I always thought that Hal was smart,
From things his friends would say,
But when he said he liked my verse,
All doubt was swept away.

Christopher Hohn

If the cover of your cookbook takes a dive into the soup,
Or the song book that you love has come apart,
Call on Lincoln Bindery's Hohn,
You can reach him on the 'phone,
And arrange for him to mend your broken heart.

B. J. Patton

When medical procedures are performed upon your body,
And payments of insurance claims appear delayed and shoddy,
Don't surrender to the company's unspeakable delay;
B. J. Patton will assist you in her quick and skillful way.

She's never apathetic or reluctant to proceed;
Whatever is your problem, she adopts it as her need.
So give her all your records and the letters you've exchanged;
Relax and stop your fretting; your relief has been arranged.

The companies all fear her when they see she's on their trail,
She always overcomes her prey; she's never known to fail.
The sight of B.J. Patton when she's just about to pounce
Brings insurance people to their knees, surrender to announce.

Jana Mason

If *Jana* rhymed with *generous* and *Mason* rhymed with
    smart,
If *practicing perfection* rhymed with *talented at art,*
If *sensitive piano playing* rhymed with *splendid health*,
A rhyme sublime in record time would nearly write itself.

Christopher Lemaistre

Christopher L., we all wish him well;
He's earned our applause and our gratitude.
He's always on board with his magical sword,
Which he wields with a genial attitude.

He handles relations with odd combinations
Of academicians assorted,
And his manner's so smooth, he can placate and soothe
Even people whose plans are aborted.

For the folks with the money, he's so friendly and sunny,
That they're eager to give us their dough;
And, with Chris's great care, our books are so square
That the auditors sing as they go.

So farewell, our Chris, whom we surely will miss,
And good luck in your future out West.
At the Ocean Pacific, may your days be terrific,
And all of your evenings the best.

The End

Dear Reader:

Your comments are invited.
I'd really be delighted.

Index of Titles

Donald M. Ginsberg

You Have the Right to Remain Silent

You have the right to remain silent
when you witness the awesome powers of nature.

You have the right to remain confused
when you consider the fundamental paradoxes of quantum
    mechanics.

You have the right to remain mystified
when you contemplate the workings of the human mind.

You have the right to remain grateful
when you think how lucky you are to be alive.

Donald M. Ginsberg

Partial Poems for the Reader to Start

...
I loved Rose Aylmer long ago,
Before you came to me.

...
On whom no mate could have a crush,
And even Ogden Nash would blush.

...
Who taught me by example, joyously,
That one can fall in love with poetry.

...
With one last heave I never shall forget,
Had risen from his bed with great regret.

...
The mean that's golden, like the sun,
If squared, will amplify by one.

...
As one you could commend,
An entertaining raconteur,
And lively to the end.

Partial Poems for the Reader to Finish

Truth resides
Where beauty hides,
Waiting to be found.
...

The rains of April fall upon the land,
Awakening the earth from deepest sleep
...

If yet these pages bring my voice to life,
When I have long abandoned earthly scenes,
...

My visual acuity leaves room for ambiguity
When looking for my glasses in the morning.
...

The string quartet that I'll not forget
Is the one that got away.
...

Night's suspended from the heavens
Like a pair of faded blue jeans,
Hanging quietly on grandma's rocking chair
...

Donald M. Ginsberg

Even at the closing of the day,

Scattered sunbeams fall and light our way.

About the Author

Donald M. Ginsberg is a professor emeritus of physics at the University of Illinois at Urbana-Champaign. In high school, a charismatic English teacher communicated her enjoyment of poetry, and encouraged him to write his first poems. He also likes playing the flute, singing, listening to classical music, trying his hand at contract bridge, and collecting rocks and minerals. He is married, has two grown children, and a twin brother (a doctor) who, like the author, enjoys making people laugh. A Fellow of the American Physical Society, the author is a winner of its Oliver E. Buckley Prize for research in condensed-matter physics.

Printed in the United States
695900002B

9 781403 323378